DIABETIC COOKBOOK
AND MEAL PLAN FOR
THE NEWLY DIAGNOSED

1000 Easy, delicious and healthy
recipes to help improve your health

SHANE RAMIRO

TABLE OF CONTENTS

DIABETIC COOKBOOK AND MEAL PLAN FOR THE NEWLY DIAGNOSED 1

1000 Easy, delicious and healthy recipes to help improve your health 1

SHANE RAMIRO 1

TABLE OF CONTENTS 3

Introduction 5

Chapter one 7

Understanding what it means of been diagnosed with type 2 diabetic 7

Chapter two 9

Meaning of diabetes 9

Types of Diabetes: 9

Common Symptoms of Diabetes: 10

Diabetes Management and Treatment: 11

Conclusion: 12

Chapter three 15

Causes of diabetes 15

Chapter four 21

Meal plan and recipes for the newly diagnosed 21

Cookbook Title: "Balanced Bites: A Diabetic's Guide to Healthy Eating" 21

Section 1: Introduction to Diabetes and Nutrition 21

Section 2: Breakfast Boosters 22

Section 3: Lunchtime Delights 22
Section 4: Dinner Dazzlers 22
Section 5: Snack Attack 23
Section 6: Sweet Endings (Desserts) 23
Section 7: Beverage Bliss 24
Section 8: Weekly Meal Plans 24
Section 9: Living Well with Diabetes 24

Chapter five **27**
The recipe 27
Recipe: Grilled Chicken Salad with Balsamic Vinaigrette 27
Ingredients: 27
Balsamic Vinaigrette: 28
Instructions: 28

Chapter six **31**
Desserts 31
Recipe: Berry and Chia Seed Pudding 31
Ingredients: 31
Instructions: 32

Conclusion: **35**

Introduction

Navigating life with diabetes can be challenging, especially for those who are newly diagnosed. The Diabetic Cookbook and Meal Plan for the Newly Diagnosed serves as a comprehensive guide, offering not just recipes but a holistic approach to managing diabetes through thoughtful nutrition. This cookbook recognizes the significance of adjusting dietary habits and empowers individuals with practical tools to make informed choices.

In the initial stages of a diabetes diagnosis, understanding what to eat and how to create balanced meals is crucial. This cookbook addresses these concerns by providing a diverse range of recipes tailored to accommodate the dietary needs of those with diabetes. From flavorful breakfast options to satisfying dinners, each recipe is thoughtfully crafted to strike a balance between taste and nutritional value.

Beyond recipes, the meal plan incorporates expert insights on portion control, carbohydrate management, and mindful eating. It aims to demystify the complexities of diabetes management, offering accessible advice for a healthier lifestyle. Whether someone is newly diagnosed or seeking to revamp their approach to nutrition, this cookbook serves as a valuable resource on the journey to better health with diabetes.

Chapter one

Understanding what it means of been diagnosed with type 2 diabetic

Being diagnosed with type 2 diabetes signifies a significant change in one's health and lifestyle. Type 2 diabetes is a chronic condition where the body becomes resistant to insulin or doesn't produce enough insulin to maintain normal blood sugar levels. This diagnosis implies a need for careful management to prevent complications.

For individuals, it means adopting a proactive role in their health, making lifestyle modifications that often include dietary changes, regular exercise, and weight management. Monitoring blood sugar levels becomes a routine, and medications may be prescribed to help regulate glucose levels.

Understanding the impact of type 2 diabetes involves recognizing the potential complications such as cardiovascular issues, kidney problems, and nerve damage. Regular check-ups with healthcare professionals become essential for ongoing assessment and adjustment of the treatment plan.

Emotionally, being diagnosed with type 2 diabetes can be challenging. It may require adapting to a new normal and overcoming potential feelings of fear or frustration. Education about the condition, its management, and the support of healthcare providers, friends, and family play vital roles in helping individuals navigate and cope with the changes associated with this diagnosis.

Chapter two

Meaning of diabetes

Diabetes is a complex and chronic medical condition characterized by elevated levels of blood glucose, commonly known as blood sugar. This results from either the body's inability to produce enough insulin or the ineffective use of insulin it does produce. Insulin is a hormone crucial for regulating glucose metabolism.

Types of Diabetes:

1. Type 1 Diabetes:
   - *Cause:* Autoimmune response destroying insulin-producing cells.
   - *Onset:* Typically occurs in childhood or adolescence.

- ○ *Treatment:* Insulin therapy is essential for managing blood sugar levels.
2. Type 2 Diabetes:
   - ○ *Cause:* Insulin resistance and inadequate insulin production.
   - ○ *Onset:* More common in adults, but increasingly diagnosed in youth.
   - ○ *Treatment:* Lifestyle changes (diet, exercise) and medications, including oral drugs and sometimes insulin.
3. Gestational Diabetes:
   - ○ *Cause:* Develops during pregnancy when the body cannot produce enough insulin.
   - ○ *Onset:* During pregnancy.
   - ○ *Treatment:* Monitoring blood sugar levels, diet modification, and sometimes medication.

Common Symptoms of Diabetes:

- Increased thirst and hunger
- Frequent urination
- Unexplained weight loss
- Fatigue
- Blurred vision

Diabetes Management and Treatment:

1. Lifestyle Modifications:
   - *Diet:* Emphasizes balanced meals, portion control, and monitoring carbohydrate intake.
   - *Exercise:* Regular physical activity aids in glucose control and weight management.
2. Medications:
   - *Oral Medications:* Improve insulin sensitivity or assist insulin production.
   - *Insulin Therapy:* Essential for Type 1 diabetes and may be prescribed for Type 2 diabetes when lifestyle changes and oral medications are insufficient.
3. Continuous Glucose Monitoring (CGM):
   - Utilizes sensors to monitor glucose levels throughout the day, providing real-time data for better management.
4. Regular Monitoring and Check-ups:
   - Blood sugar monitoring
   - A1C tests to assess long-term glucose control
   - Regular check-ups with healthcare providers for personalized guidance.

5. Complications Management:
    - Addressing potential complications, such as cardiovascular issues, kidney problems, and neuropathy.

Conclusion:

Diabetes management involves a multidimensional approach, encompassing lifestyle modifications, medication, and ongoing monitoring. With advancements in medical technology and a focus on holistic care, individuals with diabetes can lead fulfilling lives while effectively managing their condition. Regular collaboration with healthcare professionals is crucial to tailor treatment plans to individual needs and ensure optimal health outcomes.

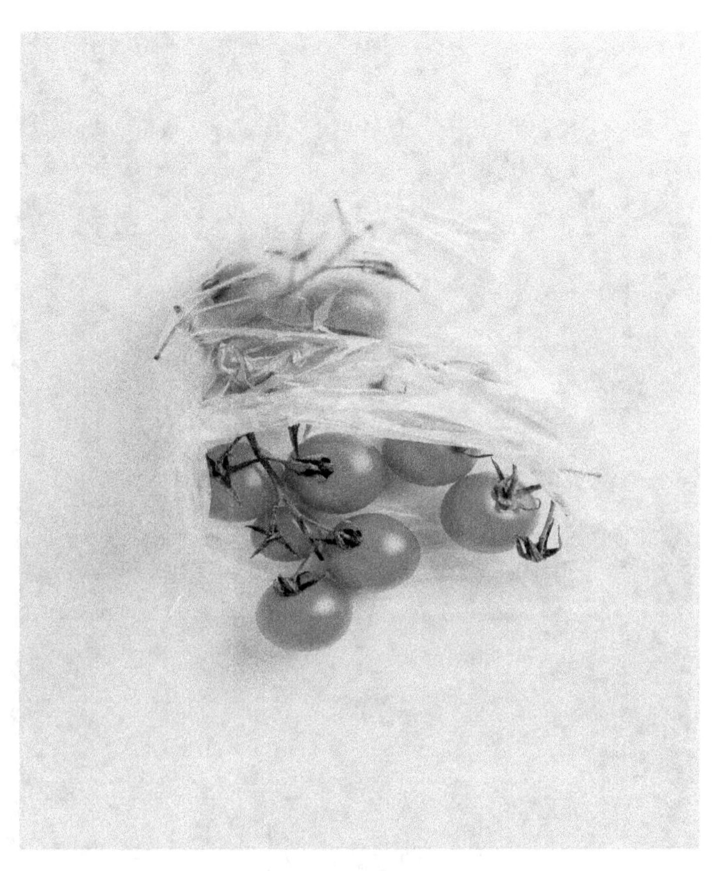

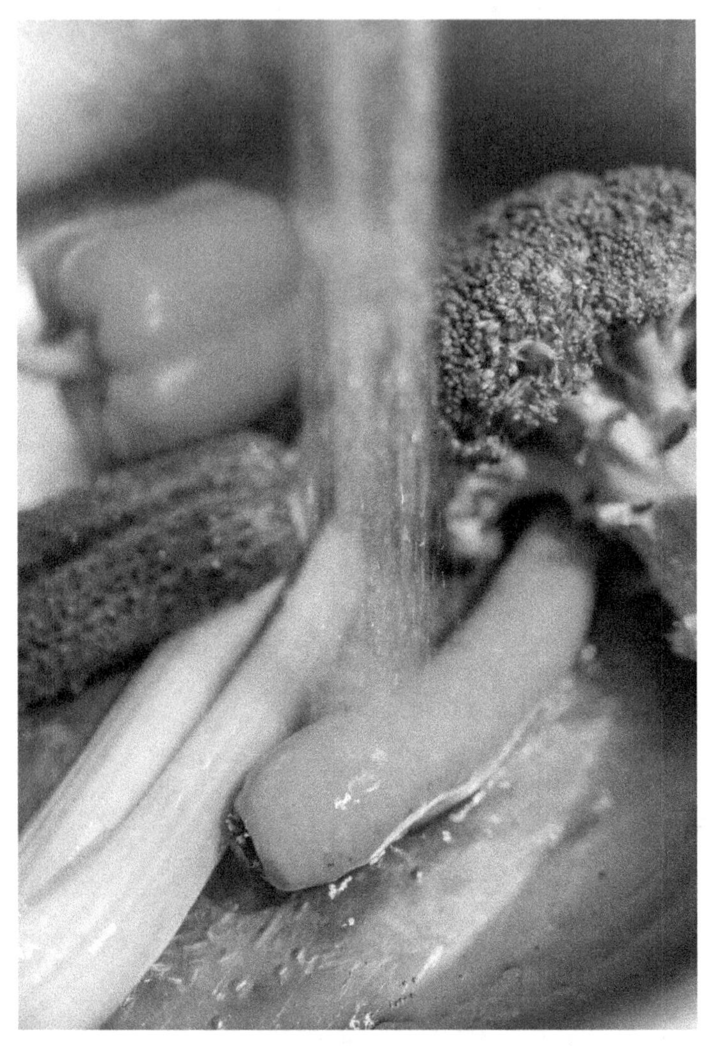

Chapter three

Causes of diabetes

Diabetes is a complex metabolic disorder influenced by a combination of genetic, environmental, and lifestyle factors. Here's a comprehensive overview of the causes:

1. Genetic Factors:
   - Family History: Individuals with a family history of diabetes, particularly first-degree relatives, have a higher risk. Specific genetic variations may contribute to susceptibility.
2. Autoimmune Factors:
   - Type 1 Diabetes: This form involves an autoimmune response where the immune

system mistakenly attacks and destroys insulin-producing beta cells in the pancreas. Genetic predisposition and environmental triggers, such as viral infections, play a role.

3. Insulin Resistance:

    - Type 2 Diabetes: The most common form is often associated with insulin resistance, where cells don't respond effectively to insulin. Genetic factors contribute, and obesity amplifies insulin resistance.

4. Environmental Factors:

    - Viral Infections: Some viruses, like enteroviruses and Coxsackie B virus, have been linked to the onset of type 1 diabetes. They may trigger an autoimmune response.

- Early Life Exposures: Adverse conditions during pregnancy or early childhood, including malnutrition or exposure to certain toxins, can influence diabetes risk.

5. Lifestyle Factors:

- Obesity: Excess body fat, especially visceral fat, is a significant risk factor for type 2 diabetes. Adipose tissue releases substances that contribute to insulin resistance.

- Physical Inactivity: Lack of regular exercise is associated with an increased risk of developing type 2 diabetes.

Exercise increases insulin sensitivity and aids in maintaining a healthy weight.

6. Dietary Factors:

   - Unhealthy Diet: Diets high in refined sugars, saturated fats, and processed foods contribute to obesity and insulin resistance. A diet low in fiber and rich in sugary beverages is linked to an elevated diabetes risk.

7. Age and Ethnicity:

   - Age: The risk of diabetes increases with age, particularly after 45. Aging is associated with changes in body composition and metabolism.

   - Ethnicity: Certain ethnic groups, such as African Americans,

Hispanics, Native Americans, and Asians, are more prone to diabetes. This may be due to genetic predisposition and lifestyle factors.

8. Hormonal Factors:

    o   Polycystic Ovary Syndrome (PCOS): Women with PCOS, characterized by hormonal imbalances, have an increased risk of insulin resistance and type 2 diabetes.

9. Gestational Diabetes:

    o   Pregnancy-related Diabetes: Gestational diabetes during pregnancy increases the risk of developing type 2 diabetes later in life for both the mother and child.

Understanding the interplay of these factors is crucial for developing effective preventive measures and personalized treatment strategies for individuals at risk of or living with diabetes. Lifestyle modifications, regular screenings, and early intervention play key roles in diabetes management.

Chapter four

Meal plan and recipes for the newly diagnosed

Creating a meal plan for individuals newly diagnosed with diabetes involves focusing on balanced, nutritious meals to help manage blood sugar levels. Here's a sample cookbook idea with recipes suitable for diabetics:

Cookbook Title: "Balanced Bites: A Diabetic's Guide to Healthy Eating"

Section 1: **Introduction to Diabetes and Nutrition**

- Chapter 1: Understanding Diabetes
- Chapter 2: Basics of Nutritious Eating for Diabetics

- Chapter 3: Reading Food Labels and Portion Control

Section 2: **Breakfast Boosters**

- Recipe 1: Quinoa Breakfast Bowl with Fresh Berries
- Recipe 2: Veggie Omelet with Avocado
- Recipe #3: Nuts & Seeds with Greek Yogurt Parfait

Section 3: **Lunchtime Delights**

- Recipe 4: Grilled Chicken Salad with Mixed Greens
- Recipe 5: Lentil and Vegetable Soup
- Recipe 6: Whole Grain Wrap with Hummus and Roasted Veggies

Section 4: **Dinner Dazzlers**

- Recipe 7: Baked Salmon with Lemon and Herbs
- Recipe 8: Quinoa-Stuffed Bell Peppers
- Recipe 9: Stir-Fried Tofu with Broccoli and Brown Rice

Section 5: **Snack Attack**

- Recipe 10: Apple Slices with Almond Butter
- Recipe 11: Greek Yogurt Dip with Fresh Vegetables
- Recipe 12: Roasted Chickpeas with Spices

Section 6: **Sweet Endings (Desserts)**

- Recipe 13: Berry and Chia Seed Pudding
- Recipe 14: Dark Chocolate Avocado Mousse

- Recipe 15: Cinnamon Baked Apples

Section 7: **Beverage Bliss**

- Recipe 16: Citrus Infused Water

- Recipe 17: Green Tea with Mint

- Recipe 18: Sparkling Berry Lemonade (Sugar-Free)

Section 8: **Weekly Meal Plans**

- 2-Week Meal Plan with Shopping Lists

- Tips for Dining Out and Special Occasions

Section 9: **Living Well with Diabetes**

- Exercise Tips and Routines

- Stress Management Techniques

- Support Systems and Resources

This cookbook combines delicious recipes with practical guidance on maintaining a healthy lifestyle for those managing diabetes. It emphasizes whole foods, fiber-rich choices, and balanced meals to help regulate blood sugar levels. Additionally, it provides tools for planning and adapting meals to individual preferences and dietary needs.

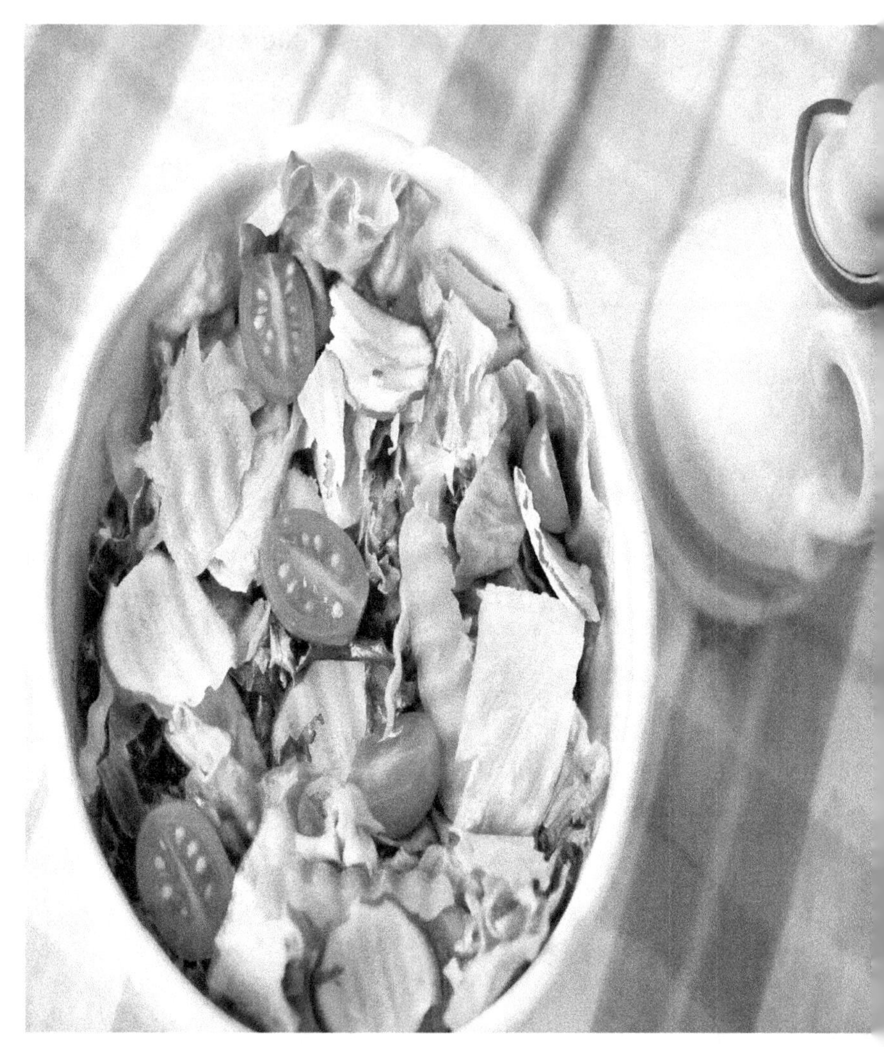

Chapter five

The recipe

Certainly! Here's a sample recipe suitable for a diabetic-friendly cookbook:

Recipe: Grilled Chicken Salad with Balsamic Vinaigrette

Ingredients:

- 2 boneless, skinless chicken breasts
- 1 tablespoon olive oil
- Salt and pepper to taste
- Six cups of mixed salad greens, (including romaine, spinach, and arugula)
- 1 cup cherry tomatoes, halved
- 1 cucumber, sliced
- 1/2 red onion, thinly sliced
- 1/4 cup feta cheese, crumbled (optional)

Balsamic Vinaigrette:

- 3 tablespoons balsamic vinegar

- 2 tablespoons olive oil

- 1 teaspoon Dijon mustard

- 1 clove garlic, minced

- Salt and pepper to taste

Instructions:

1. Preheat Grill:

   - Turn the heat up to medium-high on a grill or grill pan.

2. Season Chicken:

   - Add salt and pepper to the chicken breasts after brushing them with olive oil.

3. Grill Chicken:

   - Grill the chicken for 6-8 minutes per side or until fully cooked (internal temperature reaches

165°F or 74°C). Before slicing, let it a few minutes to rest.

4. Prepare Vinaigrette:

    o In a small bowl, whisk together balsamic vinegar, olive oil, Dijon mustard, minced garlic, salt, and pepper. Set aside.

5. Assemble Salad:

    o The red onion, cucumber, cherry tomatoes, and mixed salad greens should all be combined in a big bowl.

6. Slice Chicken:

    o Slice the grilled chicken breasts into thin strips.

7. Assemble Salad Bowls:

    o Divide the salad mixture among serving plates or bowls. Top with sliced grilled chicken.

8. Drizzle with Vinaigrette:

   - Drizzle the balsamic vinaigrette over the salad and chicken. Sprinkle with crumbled feta cheese if desired.

9. Serve:

   - Serve immediately, enjoying a flavorful and diabetes-friendly grilled chicken salad.

This recipe focuses on lean protein, fresh vegetables, and a homemade vinaigrette without added sugars, making it a nutritious and delicious option for those newly diagnosed with diabetes. Adjust portion sizes to meet individual dietary needs and consult with a healthcare professional for personalized guidance.

Chapter six

Desserts

Certainly! Here's a sample recipe for a diabetic-friendly dessert suitable for a cookbook for the newly diagnosed:

Recipe: Berry and Chia Seed Pudding

Ingredients:

- 1/4 cup chia seeds
- 1 cup unsweetened almond milk (or any preferred milk substitute)
- 1 teaspoon vanilla extract
- 1 tablespoon sugar-free sweetener (stevia or erythritol)
- 1 cup mixed berries (strawberries, blueberries, raspberries)
- Mint leaves for garnish (optional)

Instructions:

1. Prepare Chia Seed Pudding Base:

    o   In a bowl, combine chia seeds, unsweetened almond milk, vanilla extract, and sugar-free sweetener. Stir well to combine.

2. Let it Set:

    o   Cover the bowl and refrigerate the chia seed mixture for at least 2 hours or overnight, allowing it to thicken into a pudding-like consistency.

3. Assemble Individual Servings:

    o   In serving glasses or bowls, layer the chia seed pudding with fresh mixed berries.

4. Garnish:

- Add some mint leaves as a garnish for a cool touch (optional).

5. Serve Chilled:

  - Serve the berry and chia seed pudding chilled.

This dessert is rich in fiber from chia seeds and antioxidants from mixed berries, making it a diabetes-friendly option. The sweetness comes from the natural sugars in the berries, and the sugar-free sweetener adds a touch of sweetness without spiking blood sugar levels. Always tailor portion sizes to individual dietary needs and consult with a healthcare professional for personalized advice.

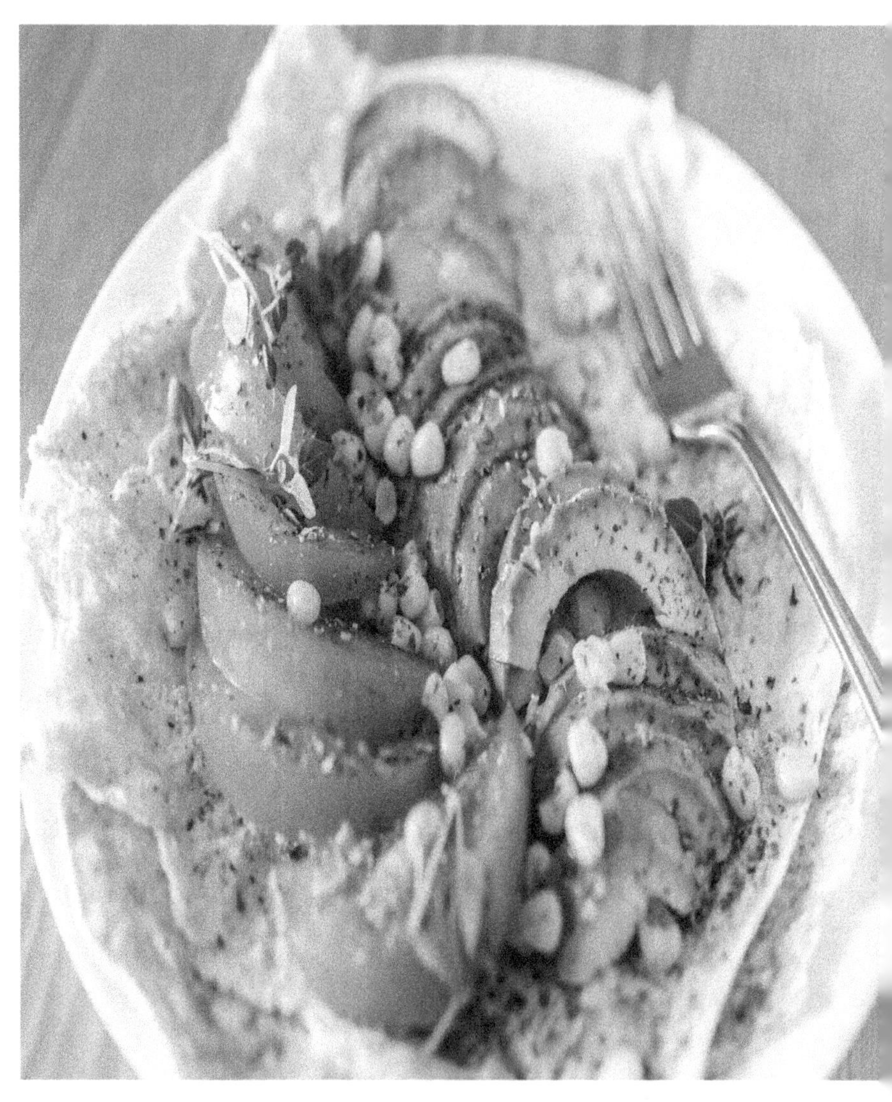

Conclusion:

Embarking on a journey to manage diabetes requires not just diligence but a flavorful commitment to nourishing the body. "Balanced Bites: A Diabetic's Guide to Healthy Eating" is not just a cookbook; it's a comprehensive guide designed for those newly diagnosed with diabetes. This collection of recipes embraces the philosophy that managing diabetes doesn't mean sacrificing taste or variety.

From energizing breakfast options like the Quinoa Breakfast Bowl to satisfying dinner delights such as Baked Salmon with Lemon and Herbs, each recipe is meticulously crafted to balance nutrition and flavor. The Grilled Chicken Salad with Balsamic Vinaigrette showcases how a well-designed meal can be both delicious and diabetes-friendly, offering a burst of freshness and protein without compromising health goals.

The Berry and Chia Seed Pudding in the dessert section exemplifies that sweetness can be achieved through natural ingredients, demonstrating that treating oneself doesn't have to mean sacrificing control over blood sugar levels. The cookbook also provides practical tools, such as weekly meal plans and shopping lists, empowering individuals to integrate healthy eating seamlessly into their daily lives.

Recognizing that living well with diabetes extends beyond the kitchen, the cookbook addresses lifestyle factors like exercise, stress management, and support systems. It's not just a compilation of recipes; it's a holistic guide aimed at fostering a balanced and sustainable approach to managing diabetes.

As individuals navigate the culinary landscape of diabetes, "Balanced Bites" serves as a trusted companion, offering not just recipes but a roadmap to a vibrant and healthful diabetic lifestyle. Here's to savoring every balanced bite and embracing a future where good food and good health go hand in hand.

www.ingramcontent.com/pod-product-compliance
Lightning Source LLC
Chambersburg PA
CBHW060904260726
48661CB00008B/3443